CARING FOR DOGS

Doris A. Freema

Table of content

INTRODUCTION

Dogs have long held a special place in our hearts as beloved companions and for good reason. Their loyalty, unconditional love, and playful nature make them not just pets but cherished members of our families. As dog owners, we have the incredible responsibility of providing them with the care and attention they need to lead happy and healthy lives. The importance of taking care of dogs goes beyond mere companionship; it encompasses numerous physical, emotional, and social benefits for both the dogs and their owners. In this discussion, we will delve into the significance of responsible dog ownership and explore the many reasons why taking care of dogs is a fundamental aspect of nurturing these incredible creatures and enhancing our own lives in the process. From the therapeutic benefits of their presence to the lessons of responsibility they teach us, let us explore the compelling reasons why dogs truly deserve the best care we can provide.

CHAPTER ONE

Types of dog food, feeding schedule, portion control

Physical care is a crucial aspect of taking care of dogs, and it starts with providing them with proper nutrition through feeding. Ensuring that your dog receives the right types of food, a consistent feeding schedule, and appropriate portion control are essential for their overall health and well-being. Here's a breakdown of each component of feeding.

Types of Dog Food:

Dry Dog Food (Kibble): Dry dog food is a popular choice for its convenience and longer shelf life. Look for high-quality brands that list meat as the primary ingredient, avoiding those with excessive fillers or artificial additives.

Wet Dog Food (Canned): Wet dog food contains higher moisture content and can be beneficial for dogs that need extra hydration or have dental issues. As with dry food, choose reputable brands with quality ingredients.

Raw Food Diet: Some dog owners opt for a raw food diet, which consists of uncooked meat, bones, fruits, and vegetables. If you choose this option, it's crucial to research thoroughly and consult with a veterinarian to ensure a balanced diet. Feeding Schedule. Establish a consistent feeding schedule based on your dog's age, size, and activity level. Most adult dogs do well with two meals per day, while puppies might need more frequent feedings. Stick to a regular feeding time to create a routine that your dog can rely on. Consistency helps prevent digestive issues and allows you to monitor your dog's appetite and health more effectively.

Portion Control: Overfeeding can lead to obesity and related health problems in dogs. Follow the recommended serving size guidelines provided on the dog food

Packaging based on your dog's weight and age. Adjust the portion size as needed, depending on your dog's activity level, metabolism, and any changes in weight.

Water Access: Ensure your dog always has access to fresh and clean water. for overall health, hydration is important. Avoid Harmful Foods, Some human foods can be toxic to dogs, such as chocolate, grapes, raisins, onions, garlic, and certain artificial sweeteners like xylitol. Avoid feeding these foods to your dog, as they can be harmful or even fatal.

Monitor Eating Habits: Keep an eye on your dog's eating habits. Changes in appetite or sudden weight loss/gain could be indicators of health issues, and you should consult a veterinarian if you notice any abnormalities. Consulting with a veterinarian is essential to determine the most appropriate diet for your specific dog based on factors like age, breed, health conditions, and activity level. Providing proper nutrition through feeding is a fundamental aspect of physical care that will contribute to your dog's overall health and happiness.

CHAPTER TWO

Importance of regular exercise, types of activities, recommended duration

Regular exercise is a fundamental aspect of caring for dogs and plays a crucial role in maintaining their physical and mental well-being. Just like humans, dogs need regular physical activity to stay healthy and happy. Physical Health Benefits: Exercise helps dogs maintain a healthy weight, preventing obesity and related health issues such as diabetes and joint problems.

It improves cardiovascular health, strengthens muscles, and enhances overall physical endurance. Mental Stimulation:

Engaging in physical activities provides mental stimulation for dogs, preventing boredom and behavioral problems that may arise from lack of stimulation.

Mental engagement during exercise can reduce stress and anxiety in dogs.

Bonding and Socialization: Exercise can be a great way for you and your dog to bond and strengthen your relationship.

Taking your dog for walks or to dog parks provides opportunities for socialization with other dogs and people, promoting well-rounded social behavior. Behavioral Benefits:

Dogs that receive regular exercise are often better behaved and less likely to engage in destructive or undesirable behaviors out of boredom.

There are various types of activities that you can engage in with your dog. The best activities will depend on your dog's breed, age, and individual preferences. Here are some popular options:

Walking: Regular walks are a simple and effective form of exercise for most dogs. It allows them to explore their environment, get fresh air, and socialize with other dogs and people.

Running or Jogging: More active breeds may enjoy running or jogging alongside you. This higher-intensity exercise is excellent for burning off excess energy.

Fetch: Playing fetch with a ball or a Frisbee can be an enjoyable and physically stimulating activity for dogs that love to chase.

Hiking: If you enjoy hiking, bringing your dog along can make it even more enjoyable. Hiking provides both physical exercise and mental stimulation from exploring new trails and scents.

Swimming: Swimming is a low-impact exercise that is gentle on joints and can be particularly beneficial for dogs with mobility issues.

Agility Training: For more active and intelligent breeds, agility training courses offer both physical and mental challenges.

The appropriate duration of exercise will depend on your dog's age, breed, and overall health. As a general guideline:

Puppies: Puppies have lots of energy, but their growing bodies are still developing. Shorter bursts of exercise, such as play sessions, should be provided throughout the day. Avoid long, strenuous activities that could put excessive stress on their joints. Adult Dogs: Most adult dogs will benefit from at least 30 minutes to 1 hour of exercise per day, depending on their breed and energy levels.

However, as dog age their need for exercise decreases but it's essential to keep them active to maintain muscle tone and joint health. Adjust the intensity and duration of exercise to accommodate their age-related changes. Always observe your dog during exercise to ensure they are not showing signs of exhaustion or distress. If you have any concerns about your dog's ability to exercise or health, consult your veterinarian for personalized advice. Regular exercise, tailored to your dog's needs, is a wonderful way to promote their overall health and happiness throughout their life.

CHAPTER THREE

Brushing, bathing, nail trimming

Grooming is an essential aspect of caring for dogs, and it goes beyond just maintaining their appearance. Here's a breakdown of three crucial grooming practices: brushing, bathing, and nail trimming

Brushing:

Brushing your dog's coat regularly helps remove dirt, loose fur, and tangles. It also stimulates the skin and distributes natural oils, which can promote a healthy coat. Long-haired breeds may require daily brushing to prevent matting, while short-haired breeds may only need weekly brushing.

Bathing:

Bathing your dog helps keep their skin and coat clean and free from dirt, debris, and odors. However, excessive bathing can strip the skin of natural oils, so it's essential not to overdo it.

The frequency of bathing depends on your dog's lifestyle, activity level, and coat type. Generally, bathing every 4 to 8 weeks is sufficient for most dogs. If your dog gets dirty or smelly between baths, you can use dry shampoo or wipes to freshen them up.

Nail Trimming:

Regular nail trimming is crucial to prevent overgrowth, which can lead to discomfort and difficulty walking. Long nails may also break or split, causing pain and potential infections.

The frequency of nail trimming depends on your dog's activity level and the surfaces they walk on. Some dogs may need their nails trimmed every 2 to 4 weeks, while others may require less frequent trimming. Be cautious not to trim

Too close to the quick (the blood vessel inside the nail). If you are unsure, ask your veterinarian or a professional groomer for guidance.

Positive Reinforcement:

Use positive reinforcement, such as treats and praise, to make grooming a positive experience for your dog. This will help them associate grooming with something enjoyable.

Use Proper Tools: Invest in high-quality grooming tools appropriate for your dog's coat type. Different brushes and combs work best for different fur textures.

Check Ears and Teeth: Regularly inspect your dog's ears for signs of infection or irritation. Additionally, maintaining good dental hygiene through regular brushing can prevent dental issues.

Watch for Skin Issues: While grooming, keep an eye out for any skin abnormalities, such as redness, rashes, or lumps. If you notice anything concerning, consult with your veterinarian.

Professional Grooming: For some dog breeds or coat types, professional grooming may be necessary. Professional groomers can handle specific grooming needs and ensure your dog receives proper care.

Grooming is an excellent opportunity to bond with your dog and monitor their overall health. Regular grooming practices will not only keep your dog looking their best but also contribute to their overall well-being and comfort.

CHAPTER FOUR

Vaccinations: importance of vaccinations, recommended schedule

Health care is a crucial aspect of responsible dog ownership, and vaccinations play a vital role in keeping dogs protected from various preventable diseases. Vaccinations are essential to safeguard not only your dog's health but also the health of other pets and humans they may come into contact with. Here's why vaccinations are important and a recommended schedule for common vaccinations:

Importance of Vaccinations:

Disease Prevention: Vaccines are designed to stimulate the dog's immune system to produce protective antibodies against specific diseases. By vaccinating your dog, you can prevent potentially life-threatening illnesses.

Community Immunity: Vaccination helps establish herd immunity within the dog population, reducing the likelihood of outbreaks and protecting vulnerable dogs who may not be able to receive certain vaccines due to health reasons.

Zoonotic Diseases: Some dog diseases, such as rabies, can be transmitted from dogs to humans. Vaccinating dogs against these zoonotic diseases helps protect both pets and people.

Affordable Prevention: Preventing diseases through vaccinations is often more cost-effective than treating serious illnesses, which can require extensive medical care.

Recommended Schedule for Common Vaccinations:

Please note that vaccination schedules may vary based on factors such as location, individual dog risk factors, and local regulations. Always consult with your veterinarian to create a customized vaccination plan for your dog. Here is a general outline of common vaccinations and their typical schedule:

Core Vaccines:

Distemper, Adenovirus (Canine Hepatitis), and Parvovirus (DA2PP or DHPP): Puppies should receive a series of vaccinations starting at 6 to 8 weeks of age and repeated every 3 to 4 weeks until they are around 16 weeks old. Adult dogs typically receive a booster one year after the last puppy vaccination and then every 3 years thereafter.

Rabies: Puppies are usually vaccinated between 12 to 16 weeks of age. Depending on the vaccine used and local regulations, the first rabies vaccination may be valid for one year or three years. Subsequent vaccinations are usually given every one to three years, depending on local laws and vaccine type.

Non-Core Vaccines:

Bordetella (Kennel Cough): This vaccine is recommended for dogs that frequently socialize with other dogs in places like boarding facilities, dog parks, or training classes. It can be administered as an intranasal or injectable vaccine, and the frequency of vaccination depends on the dog's risk of exposure.

Leptospirosis: This vaccine is recommended for dogs in areas where leptospirosis is prevalent or if the dog is at risk due to its lifestyle (e.g., exposure to wildlife or standing water). The frequency of vaccination may vary based on risk factors.

Canine Influenza: This vaccine is recommended for dogs at risk of exposure to canine influenza, such as those that visit dog parks, attend dog shows, or are boarded frequently.

Keep in mind that some vaccinations may have different intervals for booster shots, so it's essential to follow your veterinarian's recommendations for maintaining your dog's vaccination schedule. Regular check-ups with your vet provide an opportunity to discuss your dog's health and ensure they receive the appropriate vaccinations for their specific needs.

CHAPTER FIVE

Importance of veterinary visits, preventive care

Regular check-ups with a veterinarian are a crucial aspect of ensuring your dog's overall health and well-being. These visits not only allow for early detection and treatment of health issues but also play a significant role in preventive care. Here's why regular veterinary visits are essential and the importance of preventive care:

Importance of Veterinary Visits:

Early Detection of Health Issues: Regular check-ups allow the veterinarian to examine your dog thoroughly and detect any signs of health problems at an early stage. Early detection often leads to more successful treatment and can prevent minor issues from developing into serious conditions.

Vaccinations and Preventive Medications: As mentioned earlier, vaccinations protect your dog from various diseases, and regular vet visits ensure they receive timely booster shots. Veterinarians can also prescribe preventive medications for issues like heartworm, fleas, and ticks.

Customized Health Care: Each dog is unique, and regular veterinary visits enable the vet to create a customized health care plan based on your dog's age, breed, lifestyle, and individual needs.

Nutrition and Diet: Veterinarians can provide guidance on proper nutrition and diet based on your dog's specific requirements. A balanced diet is essential for your dog's overall health and can prevent nutrition-related health problems.

Behavioral Issues: If your dog is experiencing behavioral problems, a veterinarian can help identify the underlying causes and recommend appropriate training or behavior modification techniques.

Dental Care: Dental health is critical for dogs, and regular vet visits include dental examinations and cleanings to maintain good oral hygiene.

Importance of Preventive Care:

Preventing Diseases: Preventive care measures, such as vaccinations and parasite control, can protect your dog from various illnesses and infestations.

Health Monitoring: Regular check-ups allow the veterinarian to monitor your dog's health over time, making it easier to identify any subtle changes or potential issues.

Longer, Healthier Life: Providing preventive care ensures that your dog is less likely to develop preventable diseases, leading to a longer and healthier life.

Cost-Effectiveness: Preventive care is often more affordable than treating advanced illnesses or conditions that could have been avoided with proper care.

Quality of Life: By focusing on preventive care, you can enhance your dog's overall quality of life, ensuring they remain active, comfortable, and happy.

To make the most out of veterinary visits and preventive care, follow your veterinarian's recommended schedule for check-ups, vaccinations, and other preventive measures.

Additionally, always be proactive about any changes in your dog's behavior, appetite, or overall health, as early intervention is critical in maintaining their well-being. By investing in regular veterinary visits and preventive care, you can provide your dog with the best chance for a healthy and fulfilling life.

<h1 style="text-align:center">CHAPTER SIX</h1>

Brushing teeth, dental treats, regular check-ups

Dental care is essential for maintaining your dog's oral health and preventing dental issues like plaque buildup, tartar, gum disease, and bad breath.

Brush your dog's teeth with a specified toothpaste and brush, human toothpaste should not be used because it contains ingredients that are harmful to dogs. Start with short, gentle brushing sessions, and gradually increase the duration as your dog gets accustomed to the process.

Dental Chews and Toys: Provide your dog with dental chews and toys that are designed to promote dental health. Chewing on these items helps reduce plaque and tartar buildup by mechanically scrubbing the teeth.

Dental Treats: Dental treats are specifically formulated to help clean your dog's teeth while they enjoy a tasty treat. Look for treats that have a texture designed to help remove plaque and tartar as your dog chews on them.

Schedule regular dental check-ups with your veterinarian. They can perform professional dental cleanings under anesthesia, removing any stubborn tartar and assessing your dog's overall oral health.

Healthy Diet: A balanced diet contributes to overall dental health. Choose high-quality dog food that promotes dental health, and avoid excessive amounts of sugary or sticky treats that can contribute to dental issues.

Dental Treats for Dogs: When choosing dental treats for your dog, consider the following options:

Dental Chew Sticks: Dental chew sticks are usually made of rawhide or other materials that promote chewing and help reduce plaque buildup.

Dental Bones: Dental bones are typically made of natural ingredients and have a textured surface to help clean your dog's teeth as they chew.

Dental Treats with Enzymes: Some dental treats contain enzymes that can help break down plaque and prevent its formation.

Vegetable-Based Dental Treats: Some dental treats are made with vegetables like sweet potatoes or carrots, providing a healthier option for dogs with specific dietary needs.

Treats with Specific Designs: Some dental treats have unique shapes and textures, designed to reach different areas of your dog's mouth for more effective cleaning.

When choosing dental treats for your dog, consider their size, age, and specific dental needs. It's always a good idea to consult with your veterinarian to determine the best dental care routine and treats for your furry friend. Remember that dental care should be a part of your dog's overall health routine. By providing regular dental care and offering dental treats, you can help keep your dog's teeth and gums healthy, ensuring they have a happy and pain-free smile.

CHAPTER SEVEN

Importance of socializing dogs, exposing them to different environments

Emotional care is crucial for the well-being of dogs, just as it is for humans. Dogs are social animals, and providing them with appropriate socialization and exposure to different environments is essential for their emotional and behavioral development. Here are some reasons why socialization and exposure are important for dogs:

Reducing Anxiety and Fear: Socializing dogs from a young age helps them become more comfortable and confident in different situations. It can reduce anxiety and fear responses, making them less likely to develop behavioral problems related to fear or aggression. Building Positive Associations: Early and positive experiences with various people, animals, and environments can help dogs associate these encounters with positive feelings. This positive conditioning contributes to their emotional well-being and can make them more adaptable and friendly throughout their lives.

Preventing Behavioral Issues: Dogs that lack proper socialization may develop behavioral problems such as fear aggression, excessive barking, or destructive behavior. By exposing them to different environments and experiences, you can significantly reduce the risk of such issues.

Enhancing Training Success: Well-socialized dogs tend to respond better to training. When they are used to different stimuli and can remain calm in various situations, they are more receptive to learning commands and behaviors. Promoting Healthy Relationships: Socialization helps dogs learn appropriate social cues, body language, and communication skills. This is especially important when they interact with other dogs and people, ensuring they can engage in positive and safe interactions.

Preventing Isolation and Loneliness: Dogs are pack animals, and socialization allows them to feel connected and part of a larger group. This can prevent feelings of isolation and loneliness, which can negatively impact their emotional health.

Exposure to Novel Experiences: Introducing dogs to different environments, sounds, sights, and smells helps stimulate their senses and keeps their minds active and engaged. Mental stimulation is essential for preventing boredom and associated behavior problems.

When socializing your dog, it's essential to do so gradually and in a controlled manner, especially if they are young or haven't had much exposure to new situations. Start with calm and positive environments, and gradually expose them to busier and more stimulating settings.

If you have any concerns about your dog's behavior or emotional well-being, consider consulting with a professional dog trainer or a veterinary behaviorist who can provide guidance and support tailored to your dog's specific needs. Remember that emotional care is a significant aspect of responsible pet ownership and contributes to a happy and well-adjusted canine companion.

CHAPTER EIGHT

Interactive toys, puzzle games, training exercises

Physical exercise and mental stimulation are very important for dogs. Engaging their minds with interactive toys, puzzle games, and training exercises helps keep them mentally sharp, prevents boredom, and fosters a healthy and happy canine companion. Here are some effective ways to provide mental stimulation for your dog:

Interactive Toys: There are various interactive toys available for dogs, such as treat-dispensing toys and puzzle feeders. These toys require the dog to figure out how to get the treats or food, providing mental challenges and rewards for problem-solving.

Puzzle Games: Puzzle games designed for dogs often involve hiding treats or toys in compartments that the dog must manipulate or open to access the reward. These games tap into a dog's natural foraging instincts and keep them mentally engaged.

Training Exercises: Regular training sessions provide mental stimulation for dogs, as they learn new commands and behaviors. Training also strengthens the bond between you and your dog and helps reinforce good behavior.

Hide-and-Seek: Play hide-and-seek with your dog by hiding treats or toys around the house or yard. This game encourages your dog to use its sense of smell and problem-solving skills to find hidden items.

Scent Work: Engage your dog in scent work activities, such as introducing them to new scents and having them search for specific scents. Scent work is mentally stimulating and taps into their natural olfactory abilities.

Obstacle Courses: Set up a mini-obstacle course in your yard or living space using items like cones, hula hoops, and tunnels. Guide your dog through the course, encouraging them to navigate the obstacles, which provides both mental and physical stimulation.

Brain Games: There are numerous brain games designed for dogs, including interactive board games and memory games. These challenges encourage your dog to use their cognitive abilities to solve problems and earn rewards.

Social Interactions: Socializing with other dogs and people can also provide mental stimulation for your dog. Playdates with other friendly dogs or trips to the dog park allow them to interact and engage with different individuals.

Rotate Toys: To keep the novelty factor alive, rotate your dog's toys regularly. Introducing new toys and removing old ones temporarily can help maintain their interest in the toys they have.

Remember to tailor the mental stimulation activities to your dog's age, breed, and individual preferences. Dogs of different breeds and personalities may enjoy different types of mental challenges, so observe your dog's reactions and adjust the activities accordingly. Providing regular mental stimulation is a great way to keep your dog mentally sharp, happy, and content.

CHAPTER NINE

Spending time with your dog, playing, cuddling

Spending quality time with your dog is essential for building a strong bond and fostering a positive relationship. Dogs are social animals, and they thrive on companionship and interaction with their human family members. Here are some ways to spend quality time with your dog:

Playtime: Engage in interactive play sessions with your dog. Use toys like balls, Frisbees, or tug-of-war ropes to keep them physically and mentally active. Playtime is not only fun for your dog but also a great way to burn off excess energy. Training Sessions: Use training sessions as an opportunity to bond with your dog while teaching them new commands and reinforcing good behavior. Positive reinforcement methods, such as using treats and praise, can make training enjoyable for your dog.

Walks and Outdoor Adventures: Regular walks provide excellent opportunities for your dog to explore the world and experience new scents and sights. Take them to different places, like parks or nature trails, to keep the walks interesting and enriching.

Cuddling and Affection: Dogs love physical affection, and spending time cuddling and petting them helps strengthen the emotional connection between you and your furry friend. Show them love and attention through gentle touch and soothing words.

Quiet Time Together: Sometimes, all your dog needs is your presence. Sit quietly with your dog, allowing them to come to you for comfort and reassurance. This relaxed time together can be incredibly soothing for both of you.

Doggie Massage: Gently massaging your dog's muscles can be a relaxing and enjoyable experience for them. It also provides an opportunity to check for any sore spots or abnormalities on their body.

Exploring New Activities: Try out new activities together, such as agility training, nose work, or swimming (if your dog enjoys water). Exploring new activities can be mentally stimulating and create lasting memories.

Mealtime Bonding: Use mealtime as a bonding experience by hand-feeding your dog or using food-dispensing toys to make their mealtime more engaging.

Car Rides: If your dog enjoys car rides and it's safe to take them along, consider bringing them on short trips. Car rides can be exciting for dogs and offer new experiences outside their usual environment.

Photography Sessions: Capture special moments with your dog through photography. Whether it's during playtime, walks, or cuddle sessions, photographs can help preserve memories and strengthen the bond between you. Remember that spending quality time with your dog is not just about the quantity of time but also the focus and attention you give them during these moments. Every dog is unique, so observe their preferences and interests to tailor your quality time activities to suit their needs best. Your dedication to spending time with your dog will undoubtedly be reciprocated with love, loyalty, and joy from your furry companion.

CHAPTER TEN

Teaching sit, stay, come, and leash training

Training and discipline are essential aspects of responsible pet ownership. Proper training helps create a well-behaved and obedient dog, making it easier to manage them in various situations.

Start Early: Begin training your dog as early as possible, preferably when they are still puppies. Puppies have a more receptive learning capacity, and early training sets a solid foundation for future behavior.

Use Positive Reinforcement: Positive reinforcement is the most effective and humane training method. Use treats, praise, and affection to reward your dog when they perform the desired behavior. This encourages them to repeat the behavior in the future.

Teaching "Sit": Hold a treat close to your dog's nose and then slowly move it upwards, leading its head back. As their head goes up, their bottom will naturally lower into a sitting position. Once they sit, immediately give them the treat and praise.

The process should be repeated till they recognize the instruction given to them.

Teaching "Stay": Have your dog sit and then hold your hand, palm out, in front of their face while saying "stay." Take a step back and wait for a few seconds. If your dog stays in place, return to them, reward them with a treat, and praise. Gradually increase the duration and distance as your dog becomes more proficient.

Teaching "Come": Put your dog on a long leash in a safe, enclosed area. Crouch down, show them a treat, and excitedly call their name followed by "come." Gently reel them in if needed with the leash. Treat and reward when they come.

Leash Training: Leash training is essential for safe and enjoyable walks. Attach the leash to your dog's collar or harness and let them get used to wearing it indoors. Start with short walks in a quiet area, allowing them to explore while keeping the

Leash loose. If they pull, stop walking and wait until they relax the tension before proceeding.

Consistency is Key: Be consistent with your commands, rewards, and expectations. Dogs learn through repetition and predictability. Stick to the same commands and rewards to avoid confusion.

Be Patient and Positive: Training takes time and patience. Stay calm and positive during training sessions, and remember that every dog learns at their own pace.

Keep Training Sessions Short: Dogs have relatively short attention spans, especially when they're learning something new. Keep training sessions brief, and frequent, and end them on a positive note.

Seek Professional Help if Needed: If you encounter challenges during training or need additional guidance, consider enrolling in a positive reinforcement-based training class or consult a professional dog trainer. By using positive reinforcement, being patient, and providing clear and consistent commands, you can help your dog learn basic commands and leash manners effectively. The bond you create through training and discipline will contribute to a happy and well-behaved canine companion.

CHAPTER ELEVEN

Rewards and praise for good behavior

Positive reinforcement is a highly effective and humane training technique that involves rewarding and praising your dog for exhibiting desired behaviors. It works by associating good behavior with positive outcomes, making the dog more likely to repeat those behaviors in the future.

Timing is Crucial: For positive reinforcement to be effective, the reward (such as a treat) or praise should be given immediately after the desired behavior occurs. This helps the dog make a clear connection between the action and the positive consequence.

Use High-Value Rewards: Choose treats or rewards that your dog finds especially enticing. High-value treats can be more motivating for your dog and increase their enthusiasm for learning and performing the desired behavior.

Verbal Praise: Along with treats, use verbal praise to reinforce good behavior. Use a cheerful and encouraging tone to let your dog know they are doing well.

Consistency and Predictability: Be consistent in your rewards and praise. Each time your dog displays the desired behavior, reward them with the same positive reinforcement. Consistency helps reinforce the association between the action and the reward.

Vary the Rewards: While treats are common rewards, it's essential to vary the types of rewards to keep your dog engaged and motivated. Verbal praise, petting, a favorite toy, or access to an exciting activity can also be rewarding for your dog.

Keep Training Sessions Short and Fun: Training sessions should be enjoyable for both you and your dog. Keep the sessions short and end them on a positive note to maintain a positive association with training. Ignore Unwanted Behavior: When

Your dog exhibits unwanted behavior, such as jumping or barking excessively, it's best to ignore the behavior rather than punish them.

Avoid Punishment: Positive reinforcement focuses on rewarding good behavior, not punishing bad behavior. Punishment can create fear and anxiety in dogs and may lead to behavioral problems.

Be Patient: Learning takes time, and every dog learns at their own pace.

Combine Positive Reinforcement with Training Commands: Use positive reinforcement when teaching basic commands like "sit," "stay," and "come." When your dog follows the command, reward them immediately to reinforce the behavior.

 By using positive reinforcement techniques, you can create a positive and enjoyable learning environment for your dog. They will learn to associate good behavior with rewards and praise, making them more likely to repeat those behaviors in the future. Positive reinforcement not only helps with training but also strengthens the bond between you and your furry companion.

CHAPTER TWELVE

Establishing rules and boundaries, avoiding punishment-based training

Consistency is a fundamental principle in dog training and behavior management. Establishing clear rules and boundaries, while avoiding punishment-based training methods, is essential for creating a harmonious and respectful relationship with your dog.

Clarity for the Dog: Consistency provides clarity for your dog. When they understand what is expected of them and what behaviors are unacceptable, they can better navigate their environment and behave appropriately. Reliable Expectations: By being consistent in your interactions and responses, your dog knows what to anticipate from you.

This predictability fosters a sense of security and trust in your relationship. Effective Learning: Dogs learn through repetition and reinforcement. Consistency ensures that the message you're trying to convey is repeated consistently, making it easier for your dog to understand and respond to your cues and commands.

Avoiding Confusion: Inconsistent training methods or responses can confuse your dog and hinder their learning process. For example, if you allow jumping on some occasions and discourage it on others, your dog may struggle to understand when jumping is appropriate.

Building Trust and Respect: Consistency helps establish a relationship based on trust and respect. Dogs are more likely to trust and respect a leader who is consistent in their guidance and interactions.

Positive Association with Training: Consistency in using positive reinforcement and avoiding punishment-based training creates a positive and enjoyable learning experience for your dog. This encourages them to willingly engage in training sessions and obey commands.

Family and Household Unity: Consistency is especially important in multi-person households. Ensure that all family members are on the same page regarding rules and training techniques. This uniformity prevents confusion for your dog and promotes a cohesive approach to their care. Redirecting Unwanted Behavior: Rather than using punishment, redirect your dog's unwanted behavior to a more appropriate action.

Patience and Positive Reinforcement: When your dog exhibits desired behaviors, reward them with praise and positive reinforcement consistently. This encourages them to repeat those behaviors, reinforcing the training process.

Avoiding Fear and Anxiety: Punishment-based training can lead to fear and anxiety in dogs, damaging their emotional well-being and potentially causing behavioral issues.

Consistent use of positive reinforcement helps create a positive and trusting relationship with your dog. Consistency in training and setting boundaries is essential for effective communication with your dog and maintaining a healthy and respectful relationship. By using positive reinforcement techniques and avoiding punishment, you can create a positive and enjoyable learning experience for your dog, leading to a well-behaved and happy canine companion.

CHAPTER THIRTEEN

Microchipping, ID tags, keeping contact information up to date

Safety precautions are crucial to ensure the well-being and security of your dog. Identifying your dog through various methods helps increase the chances of their safe return if they ever get lost or separated from you.

Microchipping: Microchipping is a safe and permanent way to identify your dog. A microchip is a small electronic device inserted under your dog's skin, usually between the shoulder blades.

Each microchip contains a unique identification number linked to your contact information. When a lost dog is scanned for a microchip, the information is used to reunite them with their owner. Remember to register the microchip and keep your contact information up to date with the Microchip Company or registry.

ID Tags: Make sure your dog wears a collar with an ID tag that includes your phone number and any other relevant contact information. An ID tag serves as a visible and immediate way for someone to contact you if they find your lost dog. Personalized Collars:

Consider getting a personalized collar with your dog's name and your contact information embroidered or printed directly on it. This additional measure ensures that even if the ID tag is lost, there's still a way to reach you.

Keep Contact Information Up to Date: Regularly check and update your contact information with the microchip registry and on your dog's ID tags. Update your information if you move or change phone numbers.

Safe Containment: Ensure your yard or living space is properly secured to prevent your dog from wandering off or escaping. The fencing should be in good condition and tall enough to prevent jumping or climbing.

 Leash and Supervision: Always keep your dog on a leash when outside, especially in unfamiliar areas. Supervise your dog during walks and outings to prevent them from running off or getting into potentially dangerous situations. Be Prepared for Travel: When traveling with your dog, make sure they are safely secured in a carrier or harness while in a vehicle. Never leave your dog unattended in a parked car, as temperatures can rise quickly, posing a serious threat to their safety.

Training and Recall: Train your dog to come when called reliably. A strong recall command can be a lifesaver in situations where your dog might be at risk, allowing you to call them back to safety quickly.

Pet Emergency Kit: Create a pet emergency kit that includes essential supplies like food, water, first-aid items, and medications. Having this kit readily available can be invaluable in emergencies or during travel.

By implementing these safety precautions and ensuring proper identification, you can significantly reduce the risk of your dog becoming lost and increase the likelihood of their safe return in case they do get separated from you. Taking these steps demonstrates responsible pet ownership and a commitment to your dog's safety and well-being.